Treatment Guide

Understanding Nickel Allergy

By

Hywel Galen

Table of Contents

CHAPTER 1

Introduction

1.1 Understanding Nickel Allergy

Nickel allergy is a common but often misunderstood hypersensitivity reaction to nickel, a metallic element that can be found in various everyday items, from jewelry and clothing fasteners to kitchen utensils and electronics. Understanding the intricacies of nickel allergy is paramount for those affected by it, as well as for healthcare professionals, friends, and family members who want to offer support and assistance.

Nickel allergy is a delayed-type hypersensitivity reaction, meaning that it doesn't typically manifest immediately upon contact with nickel-containing objects but rather develops over time as the immune system recognizes nickel as a foreign invader. This condition primarily affects the skin but can also lead to systemic reactions in some cases. The key to comprehending nickel allergy is recognizing the underlying immune response, which can be complex and variable from person to person.

One crucial aspect of understanding nickel allergy is the prevalence of the condition. Research suggests that nickel allergy is one of the most common allergic contact dermatitides, affecting up to 15% of the general population, with a higher prevalence in females due to greater exposure to nickel through jewelry and other accessories. This high prevalence underscores the significance of raising awareness and providing effective treatment options for those affected.

Moreover, individuals often underestimate the potential severity and chronicity of nickel allergy. They may mistake the early symptoms, such as itching, redness, and swelling at the point of contact, as temporary irritation. However, without proper intervention, nickel allergy can progress to more severe symptoms, such as blistering, oozing, and the development of chronic dermatitis. In some cases, systemic symptoms can occur, leading to systemic allergic reactions. Therefore, recognizing nickel allergy as more than a minor inconvenience is crucial.

1.2 Importance of Treatment

The importance of treating nickel allergy cannot be overstated, as it can significantly impact an individual's quality of life and overall well-being. The consequences of neglecting treatment range from persistent discomfort and skin issues to potential systemic complications in severe cases.

1. *Alleviating Symptoms*: One of the primary reasons for treatment is to alleviate the often distressing and painful symptoms associated with nickel allergy. Itchiness, redness, and swelling can be not only physically uncomfortable but also emotionally distressing. When these symptoms persist, they

can interfere with daily activities, productivity, and even sleep, negatively affecting a person's overall quality of life.

2. *Preventing Progression*: Left untreated, nickel allergy can progress from localized dermatitis to chronic skin conditions. Prolonged exposure to nickel can exacerbate the problem, making it harder to manage. This progression can lead to more severe skin issues, such as open sores, chronic inflammation, and increased susceptibility to bacterial infections.

3. *Avoiding Systemic Reactions*: For some individuals, nickel allergy can extend beyond the skin and lead to systemic

allergic reactions. These reactions can range from mild hives and respiratory symptoms to life-threatening anaphylaxis. Early and effective treatment is essential to prevent the escalation of symptoms and safeguard against these potentially dangerous systemic reactions.

4. *Improving Quality of Life*: Beyond symptom relief and prevention, treating nickel allergy can improve a person's overall quality of life. It allows individuals to engage in activities without the constant worry of nickel exposure, fostering greater confidence and well-being.

5. *Long-Term Management*: Nickel allergy is often a

lifelong condition, and thus, understanding the importance of treatment is vital for long-term management. Effective treatment strategies help individuals cope with the allergy, make informed lifestyle choices, and minimize the impact of the condition on their day-to-day lives.

grasping the nuances of nickel allergy and recognizing the importance of treatment is the foundation for the comprehensive guide that follows. By understanding the condition and the significance of early, effective treatment, individuals and their support systems can better navigate the complexities of nickel allergy and take proactive steps to improve their quality of life while minimizing its impact. This guide aims to provide the knowledge and tools necessary to empower those affected by nickel allergy to manage their condition and lead healthier, more comfortable lives.

CHAPTER 2

Identifying Nickel Exposure

2.1 Common Sources of Nickel

Nickel, a versatile and durable metal, is widely used in various products and industries. Understanding the common sources of nickel exposure is pivotal for individuals with nickel allergy, as it empowers them to make informed choices to minimize contact and reduce the risk of allergic reactions.

Common sources of nickel exposure include:

1. **Jewelry**: Perhaps one of the most well-known sources of nickel exposure is jewelry, particularly inexpensive or costume jewelry. Earrings, necklaces, bracelets, and rings often contain nickel in their alloys. The prolonged contact of nickel with the skin, as is the case with jewelry, increases the risk of developing allergic reactions.

2. **Clothing Fasteners**: Many clothing items, such as zippers, buttons, snaps, and buckles, can contain nickel. These fasteners can lead to localized nickel exposure, especially in areas where the fabric directly touches the skin.

3. **Watches**: The backs of wristwatches and watchbands

are often made of nickel or nickel alloys. Wearing a watch with a nickel-containing band can lead to prolonged exposure and skin contact.

4. **Eyeglass Frames**: Frames for eyeglasses or sunglasses may contain nickel. When the frames rest on the skin, especially behind the ears and on the bridge of the nose, they can cause allergic reactions.

5. **Dental Devices**: Some dental braces, wires, and orthodontic appliances may contain nickel. Direct contact with these devices can lead to oral allergic reactions.

6. **Kitchen Utensils**: Certain kitchen utensils, cookware, and cutlery can contain nickel.

Prolonged contact while cooking or eating can result in localized exposure.

7. **Electronic Devices**: Nickel is used in various electronic devices, such as cell phones, laptops, and other gadgets. Handling these devices may lead to nickel exposure, especially if the metal is present on the surface.

8. **Belt Buckles**: Belt buckles are often made from nickel alloys. They can cause localized skin reactions where they come into contact with the skin.

9. **Coins**: Coins, especially older ones, may contain nickel. Handling coins frequently, such as cashiers or vending machine

users, can result in nickel exposure.

10. **Occupational Exposure**: Certain professions, such as metalworkers, hairstylists, and healthcare workers, may have an increased risk of nickel exposure due to their work environments.

Understanding these common sources of nickel exposure is the first step in avoiding allergenic contact. By identifying these sources in your daily life, you can take proactive measures to reduce exposure and mitigate the risk of allergic reactions. The subsequent sections will delve into methods for nickel allergy testing and recognizing allergic reactions, which are essential components of effective management.

2.2 Nickel Allergy Testing

Nickel allergy testing is a fundamental step in diagnosing and managing nickel allergy. This testing helps confirm the presence of a nickel hypersensitivity reaction and provides valuable information to guide treatment and lifestyle choices.

There are several methods for nickel allergy testing:

1. **Patch Testing**: Patch testing is the most common and reliable method for diagnosing nickel allergy. It involves applying small amounts of nickel or nickel compounds to adhesive patches, which are then affixed to the skin on the upper back. The patches are left in place for a specified duration (usually 48

hours) and monitored for any skin reactions. If a person is allergic to nickel, the area under the nickel patch will develop redness, swelling, itching, or a rash.

2. **Blood Tests**: Blood tests, such as the nickel-specific IgE blood test, can measure the levels of specific antibodies related to nickel exposure. While not as precise as patch testing, blood tests can provide supplementary information for diagnosing nickel allergy, especially in cases where patch testing may not be feasible or inconclusive.

3. **Prick Testing**: Prick testing involves applying a diluted nickel solution to the skin through a small scratch or

prick. It's primarily used when patch testing is not practical, such as in pediatric patients.

4. **Dental Testing**: In cases where dental devices are suspected as the source of nickel exposure, dental materials can be tested to confirm nickel content.

Once a diagnosis is confirmed through testing, it's crucial to communicate the results with healthcare providers, including dermatologists and allergists, to develop a personalized treatment and management plan.

2.3 Recognizing Allergic Reactions

Recognizing allergic reactions is a pivotal skill for individuals with nickel allergy. Allergic reactions can manifest in various ways, and being able to identify them early is essential for prompt treatment and mitigation of symptoms. Common allergic reactions associated with nickel exposure include:

1. **Contact Dermatitis**: The hallmark sign of nickel allergy is contact dermatitis, which is characterized by redness, itching, swelling, and a rash at the point of contact with nickel-containing objects. The skin may become blistered, scaly, or even develop open sores with chronic exposure.

2. **Systemic Symptoms**: In some cases, nickel allergy can lead to systemic symptoms, such as hives, itching in areas away from the point of contact,

gastrointestinal discomfort, and even respiratory symptoms. Severe systemic reactions, known as anaphylaxis, can occur but are rare.

3. **Oral Symptoms**: If nickel-containing dental devices are the source of exposure, symptoms can include gum inflammation, mouth sores, and a metallic taste in the mouth.

4. **Eye Irritation**: Nickel exposure through eyeglass frames can result in eye irritation, redness, and itching in the areas where the frames make contact with the skin around the eyes.

Recognizing these allergic reactions is crucial for swift and appropriate responses. Over time, individuals with nickel allergy can become more attuned to their body's responses, allowing them to take proactive steps to minimize further exposure and manage their condition effectively. Additionally, understanding the symptoms and their severity can help individuals and healthcare providers make informed decisions regarding treatment and lifestyle adjustments.

CHAPTER 3

Avoiding Nickel Exposure

3.1 Dietary Considerations

Dietary considerations play a significant role in managing nickel allergy, as some foods naturally contain nickel or can become contaminated with nickel during processing. Understanding which foods to avoid and making informed dietary choices can help reduce the risk of ingesting nickel and experiencing associated allergic reactions.

Common dietary sources of nickel include:

1. **Nuts**: Certain types of nuts, such as almonds, hazelnuts, and peanuts, are known to contain higher nickel levels. If you have a nickel allergy, it's advisable to limit or avoid these nuts in your diet.

2. **Chocolate**: Cocoa beans are known to accumulate nickel from the soil, which can then transfer to chocolate products. Dark chocolate, in particular, tends to have higher nickel content.

3. **Canned Foods**: Canned foods, especially acidic items like canned tomatoes, can be a source of nickel exposure due to the interaction between the

food and the can's metal lining. Opt for fresh or frozen alternatives whenever possible.

4. **Soy Products**: Soybeans can contain higher levels of nickel, so it's wise to moderate your consumption of soy-based foods, including soy milk and tofu.

5. **Whole Grains**: Whole grains like whole wheat, rye, and oats can have elevated nickel content. While whole grains are generally healthy, consider balancing your diet with lower-nickel grains like rice or corn.

6. **Certain Vegetables**: Some vegetables, such as spinach, lettuce, and potatoes, can accumulate nickel from the soil. Peeling and cooking these

vegetables may help reduce the nickel content.

7. **Tea**: Tea leaves, especially black tea, can contain notable levels of nickel. If you're a tea enthusiast, consider exploring herbal teas or white teas, which typically have lower nickel content.

8. **Multivitamins**: Some multivitamin supplements may contain nickel as a binding agent or in the ingredients. Check the labels and consider discussing nickel content with your healthcare provider when choosing supplements.

Understanding these dietary considerations is essential for managing nickel exposure. A dietician or healthcare provider experienced in nickel allergy can provide personalized guidance on dietary choices. For some individuals, a low-nickel diet may be recommended, which involves avoiding or limiting foods high in nickel content and opting for alternative choices that are less likely to trigger allergic reactions.

3.2 Nickel-Free Jewelry and Accessories

Avoiding nickel exposure through jewelry and accessories is a vital aspect of managing nickel allergy, as these items are among the most common sources of skin contact with nickel. Here are some key strategies for selecting nickel-free jewelry and accessories:

1. **Hypoallergenic Jewelry**: Look for jewelry labeled as "hypoallergenic." These items are designed to minimize the risk of triggering allergic reactions and are often made from materials that are less likely to contain nickel.

2. **Materials to Consider**: Opt for jewelry and accessories made from materials that are naturally low in nickel, such as stainless steel, surgical-grade stainless steel, titanium, niobium, and solid gold (14k or higher). These materials are less likely to contain nickel or release it into the skin.

3. **Coating or Plating**: Consider jewelry with a nickel-free coating or plating, which acts as a barrier between the skin

and any nickel that might be present in the base metal. However, be aware that over time, the coating may wear off, so it's important to inspect and maintain such items.

4. **Nickel Testing**: Some jewelry retailers offer nickel testing kits, which can be used to test jewelry items for nickel content. This can be a useful tool for those concerned about the nickel content of their accessories.

5. **Avoid Costume Jewelry**: Costume jewelry, often made from inexpensive metals, is more likely to contain nickel. If you have a nickel allergy, it's advisable to minimize or avoid wearing costume jewelry.

6. **Handmade or Custom Jewelry**: Handmade and custom jewelry items often allow for more control over the choice of materials. Working with a jeweler who is knowledgeable about nickel allergies can help you create custom pieces that are safe to wear.

7. **Nickel-Free Accessories**: Beyond jewelry, be cautious with other accessories like belt buckles, watchbands, and eyeglass frames. These items can also contain nickel, so seek out nickel-free alternatives when possible.

By being mindful of these considerations when choosing jewelry and accessories, you can significantly reduce your risk of skin contact with nickel. Additionally, regularly inspecting and cleaning your jewelry to prevent any nickel exposure is an essential practice for individuals with nickel allergies.

3.3 Nickel-Free Products for Personal Care

Nickel allergy doesn't stop at jewelry and accessories; it can also extend to personal care products. Many personal care items, including cosmetics, skincare products, and even toiletries, can contain nickel or nickel compounds. Identifying and switching to nickel-free alternatives is essential for managing nickel allergy and preventing skin reactions. Here are some key considerations and recommendations:

1. **Skincare Products:**

- **Check Ingredients**: Examine the ingredient lists of skincare products, especially lotions, creams, and ointments. Look for nickel-related compounds like nickel sulfate or nickel chloride. Choose products that explicitly state they are nickel-free.

- **Hypoallergenic Products**: Opt for hypoallergenic skincare products, as they are formulated to minimize the risk of triggering allergic reactions. These products are less likely to contain nickel or other common allergens.

- **Natural and Organic Options**: Consider natural or organic skincare products that use fewer synthetic chemicals, reducing the likelihood of nickel contamination. Be sure to review the ingredient list to ensure nickel-containing substances are not present.

- **Fragrance-Free**: Fragrances in skincare products may contain allergens, including nickel. Fragrance-free products are often a safer choice for individuals with sensitivities.

2. Cosmetics:

- **Nickel-Free Makeup**: Select makeup products that are specifically labeled as nickel-free. These cosmetics are manufactured with nickel-sensitive individuals in mind and are less likely to contain

nickel or nickel-based
compounds.

- **Mineral Makeup**: Some
  individuals with nickel allergies
  find mineral makeup to be a
  suitable choice, as it often
  contains fewer potential
  allergens. However, it's
  important to read the ingredient
  list carefully, as not all mineral
  makeup is nickel-free.

- **Test New Products**: Before
  applying a new cosmetic
  product to your face or body,
  perform a patch test on a small
  area of your skin to check for
  any adverse reactions.

3. Toiletries:

- **Nickel-Free Soaps**: Soap and
  body wash can sometimes
  contain nickel. Choose

hypoallergenic, fragrance-free, or gentle cleansers that are less likely to irritate sensitive skin.

- **Shampoos and Conditioners**: Haircare products can also contain nickel. Look for shampoos and conditioners labeled as nickel-free, and be cautious with hair dyes, which can sometimes contain nickel.

4. Dental Products:

- **Toothpaste**: Some toothpaste formulations may contain nickel. If you suspect your toothpaste is contributing to your nickel exposure, consider switching to a toothpaste specifically designed for sensitive teeth and gums.

5. Avoid Nickel-Containing Tools:

- Be mindful of any personal care tools you use, such as razors or tweezers, which may contain nickel. Seek out nickel-free alternatives to minimize skin contact.

When selecting personal care products, it's crucial to perform due diligence by thoroughly reviewing ingredient labels and contacting manufacturers if necessary. Additionally, don't hesitate to consult with dermatologists or allergists who can provide guidance on suitable products for your specific needs.

Managing nickel allergy in personal care products requires vigilance and a commitment to using items that are less likely to trigger allergic reactions. By being proactive and selecting nickel-free options, you can significantly reduce the risk of skin contact with nickel and better manage your condition.

CHAPTER 4

Topical Treatments

4.1 Over-the-Counter Creams and Ointments

Over-the-counter (OTC) creams and ointments can provide relief for the localized symptoms of nickel allergy, such as itching, redness, and swelling. These products are readily available at most drugstores and can be a valuable part of managing nickel allergy. Here are some common OTC treatments:

1. Corticosteroid Creams:

- *How They Work:* Corticosteroid creams and ointments are anti-inflammatory medications that can help reduce redness, itching, and swelling associated with nickel allergy reactions.

- *Application:* Apply a thin layer of the cream or ointment to the affected area of the skin. Follow the product's instructions for usage, and use it only as directed by a healthcare provider.

- *Types of Products:* There are different strengths of corticosteroid creams available over the counter. Milder strengths may be suitable for mild reactions, while stronger ones are available for more severe cases.

2. Antihistamine Creams:

- *How They Work:* Antihistamine creams contain ingredients that can help relieve itching caused by allergic reactions. These are typically used in conjunction with corticosteroid creams.

- *Application:* Apply a small amount of antihistamine cream to the affected area, following the product's instructions. Do not use these creams on broken skin or open sores.

- *Oral Antihistamines:* In addition to topical antihistamines, oral antihistamines can also be taken to alleviate itching and other allergic symptoms. However, these are typically available as separate oral medications rather than in cream form.

3. Barrier Creams:

- *How They Work:* Barrier creams create a protective layer on the skin, helping to prevent further exposure to nickel and minimize irritation.

- *Application:* Apply the barrier cream before coming into contact with potential sources of nickel. This is particularly useful for individuals who need to wear jewelry or accessories.

- *Types of Products:* Some barrier creams are formulated specifically for individuals with nickel allergies, so they may explicitly state their effectiveness in blocking nickel exposure.

4. Moisturizing Creams:

- *How They Work:* Moisturizing creams can help soothe and

hydrate the skin, which can be beneficial for managing dryness and flakiness that may occur as a result of nickel allergy reactions.

- *Application:* Apply moisturizing creams regularly, even on unaffected skin, to maintain healthy skin and minimize the risk of complications from dryness.

It's essential to follow the instructions provided with OTC creams and ointments carefully. If symptoms persist or worsen, or if you experience systemic reactions, it's crucial to consult a healthcare provider for further guidance and potentially consider prescription medications.

4.2 Prescription Medications

In more severe cases of nickel allergy or when over-the-counter treatments are insufficient, healthcare providers may prescribe specific medications to manage symptoms and reduce allergic reactions. These prescription medications are typically more potent and are often used in conjunction with lifestyle changes and avoidance strategies. Here are some common prescription medications for nickel allergy:

1. Topical Corticosteroids:

- *How They Work:* Prescription-strength corticosteroid creams or ointments are more potent than their over-the-counter counterparts and can be highly effective in reducing inflammation and itching.

- *Prescription:** These medications require a prescription from a healthcare provider, who will determine the appropriate strength and duration of use.

2. Immune Modulators:

- *How They Work:* Immune modulators, such as topical calcineurin inhibitors, can help manage allergic reactions by modulating the immune response that causes symptoms.

- *Prescription:* These medications are available only with a prescription and should be used as directed by a healthcare provider.

3. Oral Medications:

- *How They Work:* In severe cases, healthcare providers may prescribe oral medications, such as corticosteroids or antihistamines, to manage systemic symptoms or severe skin reactions.

- *Prescription:* These medications should be taken under the guidance of a healthcare provider, as they can have potential side effects and interactions.

4. Immunotherapy (Desensitization):

- *How It Works:* In certain cases, allergists may recommend immunotherapy to desensitize the body to nickel. This involves controlled exposure to increasing amounts of nickel over time to reduce the severity of allergic reactions. It is a specialized treatment and should be discussed with an allergist.

Prescription medications are an essential part of managing nickel allergy for individuals with moderate to severe symptoms or when topical OTC treatments are insufficient. However, these medications should always be used under the supervision and guidance of a qualified healthcare provider to ensure their safety and effectiveness in managing the condition. In combination with lifestyle changes and avoidance strategies, prescription medications can significantly improve the quality of life for individuals with nickel allergy.

4.3 Topical Corticosteroids

Topical corticosteroids are a class of medications commonly used to manage various inflammatory skin conditions, including allergic contact dermatitis caused by nickel allergy. These medications are available by prescription and come in various strengths, with the potency determined by the specific corticosteroid compound used. Here's a detailed look at topical corticosteroids in the context of managing nickel allergy:

How Topical Corticosteroids Work:

Corticosteroids, or simply steroids, are synthetic medications that mimic the effects of the body's natural hormones, such as cortisol. They exert anti-inflammatory and immunosuppressive effects, helping to reduce inflammation, itching, redness, and swelling, all of which are common symptoms of allergic contact dermatitis caused by nickel exposure. Topical corticosteroids work by penetrating the skin's layers and suppressing the immune response that causes these symptoms.

Types of Topical Corticosteroids:

Topical corticosteroids are categorized into classes based on their potency. These classes range from low to high potency and include:

1. **Low-Potency Corticosteroids:** These are typically used for mild cases and sensitive areas of the body. Examples include hydrocortisone and desonide.

2. **Medium-Potency Corticosteroids:** These are

used for moderate cases and less sensitive areas. Examples include triamcinolone and fluticasone.

3. **High-Potency Corticosteroids:** Reserved for more severe cases or thick, resistant skin areas. Examples include clobetasol and betamethasone.

Prescription and Proper Use:

Topical corticosteroids are available by prescription from healthcare providers, such as dermatologists or allergists. It is crucial to follow the provider's instructions for use, including the prescribed strength and application frequency. Overusing high-potency corticosteroids or using them for extended periods can lead to side effects, including skin thinning (atrophy), so it's essential to use them as directed.

Application of Topical Corticosteroids:

When applying topical corticosteroids for nickel allergy treatment:

1. **Clean the Affected Area:** Gently wash and dry the affected area before applying the medication.

2. **Apply Sparingly:** Use a thin layer of the corticosteroid cream or ointment and gently rub it into the skin until it is absorbed.

3. **Follow the Prescribed Schedule:** Apply the medication according to the schedule provided by your healthcare provider. It's

essential not to use more than directed or skip doses.

4. **Wash Hands Thoroughly:** After applying the corticosteroid, wash your hands to avoid transferring the medication to other areas of your skin or body.

5. **Avoid Contact with Eyes:** Be cautious to prevent the medication from coming into contact with your eyes, as it can cause irritation.

6. **Monitor for Improvement:** Keep track of how your skin responds to the treatment. If there is no improvement after a reasonable period, consult your healthcare provider for further guidance.

Side Effects and Precautions:

While topical corticosteroids can be highly effective, they are not without potential side effects, especially when used inappropriately or excessively. These side effects may include:

- **Skin Thinning (Atrophy):** Prolonged or inappropriate use can lead to thinning of the skin.

- **Skin Discoloration:** Some individuals may experience changes in skin pigmentation.

- **Skin Sensitization:** Long-term use can sometimes result in the skin becoming more sensitive to the medication.

- **Perioral Dermatitis:** Topical corticosteroids can trigger a specific type of rash known as perioral dermatitis in some individuals.

To minimize the risk of side effects, it is crucial to use topical corticosteroids precisely as prescribed by your healthcare provider. If you experience any adverse reactions or are concerned about side effects, discuss them with your healthcare provider.

Topical corticosteroids are a valuable component of managing nickel allergy, particularly when symptoms are severe or resistant to other treatments. When used appropriately and under medical supervision, they can provide relief from allergic contact dermatitis and improve the overall quality of life for individuals affected by nickel allergy.

CHAPTER 5

Oral Medications

5.1 Antihistamines

Antihistamines are a class of medications commonly used to manage allergic reactions, including those caused by nickel exposure. These medications work by blocking the effects of histamine, a chemical released by the immune system in response to allergens, which can lead to symptoms such as itching, redness, and swelling. Here's a closer look at antihistamines in the context of nickel allergy:

How Antihistamines Work:

Histamine is a key player in the inflammatory response that occurs during an allergic reaction. When nickel or other allergens come into contact with the skin, the immune system releases histamine, which causes the characteristic symptoms of itching, redness, and swelling. Antihistamines work by blocking the effects of histamine, thus alleviating these symptoms.

Types of Antihistamines:

There are two main types of antihistamines:

1. **First-Generation Antihistamines:** These are older antihistamines and are generally more likely to cause drowsiness as a side effect. They include diphenhydramine

(Benadryl), chlorpheniramine, and hydroxyzine.

2. **Second-Generation Antihistamines:** These are newer antihistamines that are less likely to cause drowsiness. They include cetirizine (Zyrtec), loratadine (Claritin), and fexofenadine (Allegra).

Prescription and Proper Use:

Both first-generation and second-generation antihistamines are available over the counter without a prescription, but some are available in prescription-strength formulations. Healthcare providers may recommend specific antihistamines based on the severity of the allergic reaction and individual factors.

Application of Antihistamines:

When using antihistamines for nickel allergy treatment:

1. **Follow Dosage Instructions:** Take the medication as directed by your healthcare provider or the product label.

2. **Timing:** Antihistamines can be taken either on a schedule or as needed when symptoms occur.

3. **Monitor for Drowsiness:** If you are using a first-generation antihistamine that can cause drowsiness, be cautious when operating machinery or driving.

4. **Combination Therapies:** In some cases, healthcare providers may recommend a combination of antihistamines and other medications to manage symptoms effectively.

5.2 Corticosteroids (Oral)

Oral corticosteroids are a more potent form of corticosteroid medications compared to their topical counterparts. They are typically prescribed to manage severe symptoms and systemic allergic reactions caused by nickel exposure. Here's an overview of oral corticosteroids in the context of nickel allergy:

How Oral Corticosteroids Work:

Oral corticosteroids are systemic medications that work throughout the body to suppress the immune response that triggers allergic reactions. They are highly effective in reducing inflammation and alleviating the symptoms associated with nickel allergy, particularly when symptoms are widespread or systemic.

Prescription and Proper Use:

Oral corticosteroids are available by prescription only and should be used under the guidance of a healthcare provider. They are typically prescribed for short durations to manage acute symptoms or severe allergic reactions.

Application of Oral Corticosteroids:

When prescribed oral corticosteroids for nickel allergy treatment:

1. **Follow Dosage Instructions:** Take the medication exactly as prescribed by your healthcare provider. Do not adjust the dosage without their guidance.

2. **Short-Term Use:** Oral corticosteroids are typically prescribed for short-term use to manage acute allergic reactions. Longer-term use can lead to side effects.

3. **Gradual Tapering:** In some cases, your healthcare provider may recommend a gradual tapering of the medication to prevent a rebound in symptoms upon discontinuation.

5.3 Immune Modulators

Immune modulators are a class of medications used to manage the immune system's response and inflammatory reactions, which can be beneficial in treating nickel allergy, particularly when other treatments are ineffective or when systemic symptoms are present. Here's an overview of immune modulators in the context of nickel allergy:

How Immune Modulators Work:

Immune modulators, such as topical calcineurin inhibitors like tacrolimus and pimecrolimus, work by modifying the immune response in the skin. They inhibit the activity of certain immune cells, which reduces inflammation and helps alleviate the symptoms of allergic contact dermatitis.

Prescription and Proper Use:

Immune modulators are available only by prescription and should be used as directed by a healthcare provider, typically a dermatologist or allergist.

Application of Immune Modulators:

When prescribed immune modulators for nickel allergy treatment:

1. **Apply Sparingly:** Apply a thin layer of the immune modulator to the affected skin as directed by your healthcare provider.

2. **Follow the Prescribed Schedule:** Use the medication according to the schedule provided by your healthcare provider. Do not use more than directed.

3. **Limit Sun Exposure:** Immune modulators can increase skin sensitivity to sunlight, so it's important to avoid excessive sun exposure or use sun protection measures when outdoors.

4. **Monitor for Improvement:**
   Keep track of how your skin responds to the treatment and consult your healthcare provider if there is no improvement.

Combination Therapies: In some cases, healthcare providers may recommend a combination of immune modulators with other medications, such as corticosteroids, to manage symptoms effectively.

These oral medications and immune modulators are typically reserved for more severe cases of nickel allergy or when localized treatments are ineffective. It's crucial to use these medications only as directed by a qualified healthcare provider, and any potential side effects or concerns should be discussed with them. They play an essential role in managing nickel allergy, particularly when systemic symptoms are present or when the condition is severe and widespread.

CHAPTER 6

Lifestyle Changes

6.1 Skin Care Practices

Effective skin care practices are crucial for individuals with nickel allergy. By adopting proper routines and habits, you can reduce the risk of allergic reactions and alleviate symptoms when they occur. Here's an overview of key skin care practices for managing nickel allergy:

Proper Skin Hygiene:

- **Regular Cleansing:** Cleanse your skin gently with mild, fragrance-free soap and lukewarm water. Avoid harsh cleansers, as they can strip the skin's natural barrier.

- **Moisturization:** Regularly moisturize your skin with a hypoallergenic, fragrance-free moisturizer. Well-hydrated skin is less prone to irritation.

- **Avoid Scrubbing:** Refrain from vigorous scrubbing, as it can aggravate the skin. Use a soft cloth or your hands for cleansing.

Protection from Nickel Exposure:

- **Avoid Nickel-Containing Objects:** Identify and eliminate nickel-containing items from your daily life, such as jewelry, accessories, or clothing fasteners.

- **Barrier Creams:** Consider using barrier creams on areas of the skin that come into contact with nickel, such as the earlobes if you wear earrings.

- **Nickel Testing:** If you're uncertain about the nickel content of an item, consider using a nickel testing kit to check for nickel presence.

Monitoring Skin Reactions:

- **Learn to Recognize Allergic Reactions:** Familiarize yourself with the symptoms of allergic reactions, such as itching, redness, swelling, and rashes. Early recognition is key to prompt treatment.

- **Take Action:** When you notice symptoms, use topical treatments like corticosteroid creams or antihistamines as recommended by your healthcare provider.

6.2 Clothing Choices

Clothing choices play a significant role in minimizing skin contact with nickel. Selecting the right garments and making informed choices can help reduce the risk of allergic reactions. Here are some clothing-related considerations:

Fabric Selection:

- **Choose Nickel-Free Fabrics:** Opt for clothing made from fabrics that are less likely to contain nickel. Natural fibers like cotton and silk are typically safe choices. Avoid synthetic fabrics that might contain traces of nickel.

- **Wash New Clothing:** Before wearing new clothing items, wash them to remove any potential contaminants or irritants.

Avoiding Nickel-Containing Fasteners:

- **Check Labels:** Examine clothing labels for information about nickel-containing hardware, such as buttons, snaps, zippers, and clasps. Avoid items with nickel fasteners.

- **Modify Clothing:** If you have a clothing item you love but it contains nickel fasteners, consider replacing them with nickel-free alternatives.

- **Wear Protective Barriers:** If a garment has nickel fasteners, wear a protective barrier like a hypoallergenic undershirt to prevent direct contact with the skin.

6.3 Home Environment Modifications

Modifying your home environment is another essential aspect of managing nickel allergy. By reducing potential sources of nickel exposure in your living spaces, you can create a safer and more comfortable environment. Here are some key home environment modifications:

Kitchen and Dining:

- **Choose Nickel-Free Cookware:** opt for cookware and utensils made from stainless steel or other nickel-free materials to avoid nickel leaching into your food.

- **Avoid Nickel-Containing Kitchen Tools:** Use utensils and appliances that are nickel-free, especially if you have a history of reactions while cooking.

Bedroom and Personal Space:

- **Nickel-Free Accessories:** Ensure that your bed frame, headboard, and other bedroom accessories are nickel-free.

- **Jewelry Storage:** Store jewelry in containers or storage solutions that prevent direct skin contact.

Bathroom and Personal Care:

- **Nickel-Free Razors and Toiletries:** Choose personal care items, including razors, toothbrushes, and other accessories, that are nickel-free.

- **Nickel-Free Bathroom Fixtures:** If possible, use nickel-free fixtures in your bathroom to avoid skin contact.

Home Maintenance:

- **Choose Nickel-Free Fasteners:** When making repairs or renovations in your home, request nickel-free fasteners for your furniture, cabinets, and fixtures.

- **Carpets and Flooring:** Consider flooring and carpeting that do not contain nickel or have nickel-containing components.

Making these modifications in your home environment can contribute to a safer and more comfortable living space for individuals with nickel allergies. By being proactive and informed, you can create a supportive environment that complements other aspects of nickel allergy management, such as avoidance strategies and treatment options.

CHAPTER 7

Managing Allergic Reactions

7.1 First Aid for Nickel Allergy Reactions

Managing allergic reactions to nickel, especially when they occur, is a crucial part of living with a nickel allergy. Knowing how to provide first aid and alleviate symptoms can make a significant difference in your comfort and well-being. Here's an overview of first aid measures for nickel allergy reactions:

Recognizing Allergic Reactions:

- Familiarize yourself with the common symptoms of nickel

allergy, such as itching, redness, swelling, and rashes.

- Early recognition of symptoms is essential for timely intervention.

Immediate Actions:

- If you suspect you've had skin contact with nickel and start experiencing symptoms, remove the source of exposure immediately.

- Gently cleanse the affected area with mild, fragrance-free soap and water to remove any residual nickel.

- Apply a cold compress to alleviate itching and reduce redness and swelling.

Topical Treatments:

- If you have topical treatments prescribed by your healthcare provider, apply them as directed. These may include corticosteroid creams or antihistamine creams.

- Avoid scratching, as it can worsen symptoms and increase the risk of infection.

Oral Antihistamines:

- If itching and discomfort persist, you can take an oral antihistamine as directed. These are available over the counter and can help alleviate symptoms.

Consult a Healthcare Provider:

- If symptoms do not improve or if you have concerns about your allergic reaction, contact your

healthcare provider for
guidance.

7.2 Emergency Response and Anaphylaxis

While nickel allergy reactions are
often localized to the skin, in some
cases, individuals can experience
more severe reactions that may
involve multiple systems, a condition
known as anaphylaxis. Anaphylaxis is
a life-threatening medical emergency
that requires immediate attention.
Here's what you need to know about
managing anaphylaxis due to nickel
allergy:

Recognizing Anaphylaxis:

Anaphylaxis is characterized by a
rapid and severe onset of symptoms,
which may include:

- Difficulty breathing or wheezing

- Swelling of the face, lips, or tongue

- A sudden drop in blood pressure

- Rapid or weak pulse

- Loss of consciousness

- Severe nausea, vomiting, or diarrhea

- Hives or widespread skin redness

Immediate Actions for Anaphylaxis:

If you suspect anaphylaxis due to nickel exposure, take the following immediate actions:

- Dial emergency services (911 or the appropriate emergency number) for assistance.

- If you have an epinephrine auto-injector (e.g., EpiPen), use it as directed by your healthcare provider or as you've been trained to do.

- If you are with someone who is experiencing anaphylaxis, administer their epinephrine auto-injector if they have one and are unable to do so themselves.

- Lie the person down and elevate their legs to improve blood flow to the heart.

- If they are unconscious and not breathing, begin cardiopulmonary resuscitation

(CPR) if you are trained to do so.

After Anaphylaxis:

Even if the person's condition improves after administering epinephrine, it is essential to seek immediate medical attention at a hospital. Anaphylaxis can have delayed or secondary reactions that require further treatment and monitoring.

Managing anaphylaxis due to nickel allergy requires quick and effective response. Individuals with a history of severe allergic reactions should carry an epinephrine auto-injector and be trained on how to use it. It's also important to wear a medical alert bracelet or necklace to inform healthcare providers of your nickel allergy and the risk of anaphylaxis.

Recognizing the signs of an allergic reaction, knowing how to provide first aid for localized symptoms, and being prepared to respond to anaphylaxis are vital aspects of managing nickel allergy and ensuring your safety. It's essential to be proactive, informed, and prepared to handle various situations that may arise as a result of nickel allergy.

CHAPTER 8

Consultation with a Healthcare Provider

8.1 Finding the Right Specialist

Finding the right healthcare specialist is essential for effectively managing nickel allergy. While general practitioners can provide valuable guidance, you may benefit from consulting with specialists who have expertise in allergies and dermatology. Here's how to find the right specialist:

1. Allergist/Immunologist:

- Allergists are specialists in the diagnosis and treatment of allergies, including nickel allergy.

- Consider seeking an allergist for comprehensive evaluation, diagnosis, and treatment options.

2. Dermatologist:

- Dermatologists specialize in skin conditions and can be particularly helpful if you experience severe skin reactions due to nickel allergy.

- They can recommend topical treatments and strategies for managing skin symptoms.

3. Allergy Clinic:

- Some larger medical centers and hospitals have dedicated allergy clinics staffed by a team

of allergists and other
specialists.

- An allergy clinic can provide
  comprehensive care and testing
  for nickel allergy.

4. Recommendations:

- Ask your primary care
  physician for recommendations
  on allergists or dermatologists
  in your area.

- Seek referrals from friends or
  family members who have
  received care for allergies or
  skin conditions.

8.2 Preparing for Your Medical Appointment

Preparing for your medical
appointment with a healthcare

provider is important for ensuring a productive and informative visit. Here are steps to help you get the most out of your appointment:

Documentation:

- Compile a list of your symptoms, including when they first appeared and their severity.

- Document any potential triggers, such as specific items or activities that coincide with your symptoms.

- List any medications you are currently taking, including over-the-counter and prescription drugs.

Questions:

- Prepare a list of questions and concerns you have about your nickel allergy, such as treatment options, lifestyle modifications, and symptom management.

Medical History:

- Provide a detailed medical history, including any allergies, skin conditions, or chronic illnesses.

Testing and Diagnosis:

- If you've had any previous allergy testing or skin patch tests related to nickel, bring the results and any relevant medical records.

Symptom Diary:

- Consider keeping a symptom diary leading up to your appointment. Document when symptoms occur, what you were doing, and any potential triggers.

8.3 Questions to Ask Your Doctor

During your medical appointment with a healthcare provider, it's essential to ask questions and seek clarification on any concerns you may have about your nickel allergy. Here are some questions to consider asking:

General Questions:

1. What is the cause of my allergic reactions to nickel?

2. Are there any specific tests to confirm a nickel allergy diagnosis?

3. What treatment options are available for nickel allergy, and

which one would be most suitable for me?

4. Are there lifestyle changes or avoidance strategies that can help reduce my exposure to nickel?

5. What are the potential risks and benefits of the recommended treatment options?

Treatment and Medication:

6. What over-the-counter treatments are effective for managing nickel allergy symptoms?

7. Are there prescription medications, such as corticosteroids or antihistamines, that can help with symptom management?

8. How should I use any prescribed medications, and what potential side effects should I be aware of?

Lifestyle Modifications:

9. What clothing choices, personal care products, and accessories should I avoid to reduce nickel exposure?

10. Are there any specific skin care practices I should follow to minimize symptoms?

Testing and Monitoring:

11. How often should I undergo testing or check-ups to monitor my condition and treatment progress?

12. What signs or symptoms should I be alert to that might indicate

a need for immediate medical attention?

Emergency Preparedness:

13. Do I need an epinephrine auto-injector for severe allergic reactions, and if so, how should I use it?

Follow-Up:

14. What is the recommended follow-up plan to evaluate the effectiveness of treatment and make any necessary adjustments?

15. Can you provide written instructions or a treatment plan for managing nickel allergy?

Don't hesitate to ask your healthcare provider any additional questions or concerns that are specific to your condition and circumstances.

Effective communication with your provider is key to ensuring you receive the most appropriate care and guidance for managing nickel allergy.

CHAPTER 9

Alternative and Complementary Therapies

9.1 Acupuncture

Acupuncture is an alternative therapy that involves the insertion of fine needles into specific points on the body to promote healing and balance. While acupuncture is primarily used for various health conditions, it is not considered a mainstream treatment for nickel allergy. However, some individuals explore alternative therapies like acupuncture to manage allergy symptoms, and it may provide relief for certain symptoms such as itching and skin inflammation.

Important Considerations:

- If you're interested in acupuncture as a complementary therapy for nickel allergy, consult with a licensed acupuncturist who has experience in treating allergic conditions.

- Discuss your nickel allergy and its symptoms with the acupuncturist to determine if acupuncture might be a suitable option for you.

- Keep in mind that acupuncture is not a replacement for standard medical treatment, including avoidance strategies and prescribed medications.

9.2 Herbal Remedies

Herbal remedies, which include the use of plant-based substances, are sometimes considered as complementary treatments for allergies. There is limited scientific evidence to support the use of herbal remedies for nickel allergy. Some herbs may have anti-inflammatory or antihistamine properties, which could potentially provide relief from allergy symptoms.

Important Considerations:

- Consult with a qualified herbalist or healthcare provider before using herbal remedies to ensure they are safe and appropriate for your condition.

- Be aware that herbal remedies can interact with other medications and may have side effects or allergic reactions of their own. Share your full medical history and current medication list with your healthcare provider.

- Keep in mind that the effectiveness of herbal remedies can vary from person to person, and they are not a guaranteed or primary treatment for nickel allergy.

9.3 Dietary Supplements

Dietary supplements, such as vitamins and minerals, are sometimes explored as complementary treatments for allergies and related symptoms. While supplements can support overall health and immune function, they are not a direct treatment for nickel allergy. Here are some considerations when it comes to dietary supplements:

- **Vitamin C:** Some individuals take vitamin C supplements for their potential anti-inflammatory and antihistamine properties. Adequate vitamin C intake can support overall immune health.

- **Quercetin:** Quercetin is a flavonoid found in various foods, and it is believed to have antihistamine and anti-inflammatory effects. Some people take quercetin supplements to manage allergy symptoms.

Important Considerations:

- Consult with a healthcare provider before starting any dietary supplement regimen to ensure they are safe and appropriate for your individual needs.

- Supplements are meant to complement a balanced diet, not replace it. Ensure you maintain a healthy diet rich in nutrients to support your immune system.

- Be aware that while supplements may have potential benefits, their effectiveness can vary, and they should not be considered a primary treatment for nickel allergy.

It's essential to approach alternative and complementary therapies for nickel allergy with caution and in consultation with healthcare professionals. These therapies should not replace standard medical treatment and avoidance strategies, but they may offer additional relief or support for some individuals. Always prioritize the guidance and recommendations of your healthcare provider in managing nickel allergy.